Stress-Free Parenting in 12 Steps

Stress-Free Parenting

in 12 Steps

Christiane Kutik

Floris Books

Translated by Matthew Barton

First published in German as *Erziehen mit Gelassenheit*
by Verlag Freies Geistesleben in 2009
First published in English by Floris books in 2010
© 2009 Verlag Freies Geistesleben & Urachhaus GmbH, Stuttgart
English version © Floris Books 2010

British CIP Data available
ISBN 978-086315-762-2
Printed in Great Britain
by Bell & Bain Ltd., Glasgow

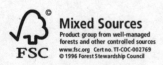

Mixed Sources
Product group from well-managed
forests and other controlled sources
www.fsc.org Cert no. TT-COC-002769
© 1996 Forest Stewardship Council

Contents

Introduction

The birth of a child is a time of great joy and delight. Parents feel on top of the world. But if you ask them how they feel a few weeks or months later, the picture is often somewhat different, with tired and tearful mothers at their wits' end: 'I can't stop for a moment. My child takes all my time and energy. I have no time to myself any more. I'm completely exhausted.'

These days, increasingly, parents are finding daily life with young children difficult. They feel pressured to get everything right and be liked by their children. When, precisely because of these pressures, they get stressed, the initial joy of having children quickly evaporates. Yet they long to steer their daily life into calmer waters, to feel less tired, so the family can enjoy their time together.

This book shows how we adults can set course for a calmer existence, in twelve steps that will help to remove stress and improve our quality of life.

An underlying structure gives family life solidity and direction. This involves clarity of *roles, respect, rules* and *rhythm.* When children see that parents are clear about their role, unequivocal and reliable; where respect and adherence to certain rules are practised and required; where there is a clear rhythm to the day and firm, reliably repeated times for certain activities, the most tiring stress factors fade. That's the foundation.

We can enhance quality of life by marking transitions in the day with enjoyable, regularly recurring *rituals,* and by being *responsive* to children. We must also give them loving support, *reassurance* and *room* to grow so that they feel accepted. In this way they learn to develop their own capacities. Consciously created moments of *repose* and times for *religion* and spiritual connection also enhance quality of life. And times of *regeneration* and *reflection* are likewise important for parents to renew and refresh themselves.

Being a parent involves showing the way — something our children call on us to do, day in, day out. The more challenging they are, the clearer this call to us is. Our task is to lead from the front and to give children what they need so much today: the space to grow through their own achievements, as well as protection, security and love. Implicit in love are courage, taking a stance and making a stand, along with sometimes putting up with a degree of frustration rather than always trying to please our children. Friction creates warmth.

So come with me on this journey, in which pleasure and happiness can soon regain their central place in family life.

Christiane Kutik

1. Roles

On a pavement beside a busy street. For the past five minutes parents have been asking their two-year-old, 'Would you rather go in the buggy or do you want to walk?' The little boy keeps getting up and down, and the parents are at a loss: 'Come on now, make up your mind! Which would you like to do? Do you want to walk or shall we push you?' The boy grimaces and then starts to cry. 'Now there's really no need to cry,' says the father. 'We've been asking you what you want to do.'

  Questions, questions, questions: a lot of time, words and energy. The parents are clearly irritated because their son isn't giving them a straightforward answer. But can such a small child really do that?

Asking children to make decisions

This little boy isn't crying because of the buggy, but because too much is being asked of him. At the age of two he can't yet decide things as an adult can. Children can't even do this at four or five. Anna Jean Ayres, among others, has demonstrated this in her seminal research, writing, 'Higher intellectual capacities only develop after the age of seven.'[1]

Children are not partners

Children are not decision-makers, partners or friends, but are in the process of gradually developing their own capacities. For this process to succeed they need — as an apprentice needs a master — their parents to lead, guide and reflect back to them.

It is therefore vital to avoid elevating a child into a position of power for which he is not yet ready. Don't ask him whether he'd rather do this or that. Don't endlessly explain things to him and try to persuade him, even if it is fashionable nowadays to thrash out any and every issue with the smallest infant. As we can see, this always leads to more stress for everyone involved. Adults get annoyed if a child doesn't know what he wants. And the child grows nervous, uncertain and 'difficult' if he doesn't feel secure with adults. To reach our goal of 'stress-free parenting,' the parents' clear sense of their role is the primary, essential thing.

Clarity of roles

It is our job to clearly accept and acknowledge our role of responsibility as caregivers instead of always asking a child what he wants. Unlike a child, we have a life's worth of experience that can help us assess a situation and offer guidance. If we do so, we give the child what he really needs: a sense that the grown-ups know what should be done. This is active love, which gives him sure ground beneath his feet and a sense of security. It means that the child doesn't have to keep expending his life forces on small things. Instead he can use them for his own role of being a child and developing, taking his lead from our example.

Trying to please the child

'But I ask my child because I want him to be happy,' is a phrase we often here. Let's just observe, though, how continually asking a child whether he wants one thing or another affects him. Does this make him relaxed, calm or happy? No. He is much more likely to send out emergency signals in response, such as shouting, crying and making a fuss. Why is this?

Small children live in the moment, and are as inconstant as a butterfly: something glitters, something else moves, something gives off a scent; their senses are always open to the manifold impressions surrounding them that spark their interest. Children naturally want everything. That's why we're asking for trouble if we expect clear decisions from them.

'What would you like for lunch today?' a mother asks her three-year-old in the supermarket. 'Would you like broccoli? We could also have noodles. Or would you rather have pancakes?' Back and forth it goes, becoming increasingly stressful. 'Broccoli,' the child says at last.

The mother buys it and cooks it. But at lunchtime there's a fuss again because Luke pushes his plate away. 'But you said you wanted it,' complains the mother, and is irritated because her child is being so 'difficult' again.

Magic armour

We can avoid such irritation if we grasp one basic thing: a child is a child and not a friend. To a mate of mine I might say, 'Hey, I'd like to cook a meal for you — what do you feel like eating?' If he replies that he wants, say, 'Sausages and mash,' we can be sure he'll enjoy it when it arrives. Children aren't like this, so we should let them be children and have the courage to decide for them instead of asking for their approval and agreement in every decision. Jacques Lusseyran describes vividly how deeply a child longs for guidance.[2] He describes the 'joy of my childhood' as being 'that marvellous sense of living not yet on one's own, but leaning body and soul on others who accept the charge.' He calls this the 'magic armour which, once put on, protects for a lifetime.'

All children need this 'magic armour' — and we give it to them when we take clear responsibility. On a ship, after all, the captain, not the deckhand, decides which direction to sail in.

What if my child doesn't like the food I give him?

'What should I do if I don't ask my child what he'd like to eat and he says, "I don't like it"?'

Persist in acting as an example yourself, because children take their lead from us. Cook tasty meals. It doesn't have to be expensive; simple meals are easily made, such as a lovely plate of golden-yellow saffron rice. On no account send children out of the kitchen because that 'speeds things up' (see Chapter 8, p.90), but instead include them in cooking from a young age. They can wash potatoes, cut vegetables, stir salad dressing. In this way they will be involved with all their senses, smelling the appetizing aromas when, for instance, onions are sizzling in butter. This will get their digestive juices flowing. Then arrange things nicely: a lovingly laid table simultaneously awakens the child's aesthetic sense. And then, during the meal, maintain your example by eating with pleasure yourself: 'Mm, the salad dressing tastes lovely today — delicious with fresh herbs and lemon juice.'

But what if the child still says that he doesn't like it?

Children often say this to see what will happen. If they see that whenever they say this it upsets the adults, it will give them an intriguing sense of their own power. A little humour solves the problem better than showing hurt or upset: 'I'm sorry you don't like it,' and then keep eating yourself with enjoyment. Don't even bother trying to persuade them to try a little. Children take their lead from what we do ourselves, the example we give, and we can trust in this. What best motivates our children is not words and arguments but our own example.

In a subway I once saw these words written on the wall: 'We don't need to bring up our children, they copy everything we do!' True indeed!

Children need clarity

Children accept the adult who is clear in his role, and clearly states what is to happen and how. It's astonishing how quickly they grasp what you mean.

On a tram journey, a father gets on through the first door down from the driver's cab with his three-year-old in a buggy. The boy climbs out of the buggy and hammers on the driver's cab. The father says, 'Would you like a biscuit?' The boy glances at him then hammers again, making an impressive racket. The father says, 'Would you like a drink?' He passes the child his drinking bottle. But the child still goes on hammering. The driver comes out of his cab, looks the child in the eye and says, 'Right, be quiet now, otherwise I can't drive the tram.' The child stares up at the man with wide eyes and is immediately still.

Instruction not diversion

Why does the child accept what the tram driver says? He does something very important, stating what he expects of the child at that moment: 'Right, be quiet now ...' This is a clear instruction. And this is what children need because they can't tell what, where, when and how something is right or not. Instruction not diversion. Here the driver gives the instruction. It is not just his words that are effective, but his whole presence and bearing. There is no trace of uncertainty, and his look and gestures speak a clear language. The child knows immediately what the driver expects — and this is the important thing. Children want to know what is expected.

Clarity of roles is the key

We must get away from the false idea that parents who take a clear role are being domineering. Not doing this is actually less caring.

Children are children, and are on the way to learning at all levels, to acquiring their own capacities. It is quite clear that they are not our partners, nor our bosses, nor decision-makers; nor are parents friends or long-term wish-fulfillers.

What are we then? As parents we are learning to be parents. To begin with we have little experience; we make mistakes and blunders. That's part of the learning curve. But we should never forget that as parents we are examples whether we wish to be or not. We are, as it were, permanently on-stage. And children reflect everything: if we are unsure of ourselves as adults, this unsettles them. If we have poise, this gives them security.

Practising clarity of roles

Clarity of roles begins in your mind. What's important is to recognize how necessary this clarity is, how it helps us to avoid cul-de-sacs in childcare.

The moment we take courage as adults to take the lead, we can free ourselves from the 'crazy circus' of daily stress. Our natural role is to lead and to decide what is happening: when, where and how.

We can practise this clarity and remind ourselves of it, for instance, by writing 'Clarity of roles!' on the mirror, in a notebook or on a pinboard. Put it up wherever you often look, so that you don't keep making a rod for your own back and get irritated when a child fails to understand what's expected.

Clarity of roles in 5 steps

'Our child is really difficult: she never does what she's supposed to,' said the mother of four-year-old Joanna. 'For example, in the evening, when I put on her pyjamas, she shouts and calls out "stupid Mum" and undresses again immediately. It's the same every day. I have to resort to shouting back — then she'll do it. But I feel bad afterwards and have a bad conscience.'

Whenever there are difficulties because a child refuses to do something, does not 'listen' or runs away, the first thing we need to do is be very clear. The following five rules are very helpful:

1. Pay complete attention — no multi-tasking — but be completely present yourself.
2. Address the child by name.
3. Eye contact: look your child in the eye. According to a Chinese proverb, 'The gaze is the second spine.'

4. State clearly what you want: tell your child exactly what this is about.
5. Keep your eye on the ball: stay with this until you have got there.

Joanna's mother decides not to let her child manipulate her any more. She tries the following in the evening, when it's time to put on pyjamas:

1. She does no other tasks, for instance, leaving the washing-up for now. She does not answer the telephone. She is completely present with her child. Her sole focus now is that her daughter should put on her pyjamas without a tantrum.
2. She addresses the child by name. We often overlook this and call out something impersonal, but saying someone's name calls on their full attention. Joanna notices that Mum really means her.
3. Eye contact is also important; it is not for nothing that the eyes are called the 'windows of the soul.'
4. Then a clear statement of what is wanted: 'Joanna, it's time to put on your pyjamas.' Joanna wants to run away: that's what she's used to, ignoring what is asked and running off. But now? Today her mother has decided to keep a clear focus. What does she do?
5. She keeps her eye on the ball: 'Joanna, look at me please.' The child keeps looking away. 'I'm waiting.' Why is it so important that eye contact occurs, even briefly? We can experience this for ourselves: eye language connects — a momentary spark of contact is enough. Children also feel this, because they often try to avoid our eyes. But now Joanna returns the look, and that's the important thing. Now she has understood, and she puts on her pyjamas without a fuss.

It actually works!

'The five steps really do work,' says a mother at our next meeting. 'It even worked with my fifteen-year-old teenager. For weeks it's been annoying me that he turns up his music so loud, so I tried to tackle it with the five steps. In the middle of the day, before he disappeared into his room, I took him aside. The first thing I noticed was how rarely I actually call him by name. I found it quite strange to say, "Thomas ..." And the eye contact — I never really paid any attention to it before. Then I said what was bothering me. I'd really thought about this beforehand: what do I really want? So I told him very clearly, "Thomas, please turn your music down lower than yesterday, otherwise it gives me a headache and I can't concentrate on anything." He said, "That's fine. Anything else?" After a while he put his head out of his door and asked, "OK?" "Yes," I replied, "that's great. Thanks Thomas."'

Helping children to grow

Children are precious. If we do the right thing for them by leading the way as adults, taking responsibility and setting a clear example, daily family life becomes more relaxed.

> *To bear fruit a tree needs:*
> *air, good earth, the sun and rain.*
> *To unfold and develop a human being needs:*
> *food, protection and a heart*
> *open with love,*
> *another who helps him grow.*

Ute Craemer

2. Respect

A mother is with her four-year-old son on the underground. The little boy wants something. The mother says, 'Not now!' At this, the boy kicks out and hits the mother's shinbone with his foot. She briefly flinches but says nothing. Not a word or a look. As though nothing had happened, she gets out at the next stop with her child.

My child often lashes out

Children hitting their own parents is an urgent problem today.

'But it's quite normal,' says one mother, 'they all do it nowadays.'

Another says, 'It doesn't bother me, but I don't want my child hitting other people.'

A young sibling, for instance, should be protected from this: 'My two-and-a-half-year-old son continually throws all kinds of things around, intentionally aiming at people, for instance myself and my husband. He also often lashes out. We're having another child in three weeks, and we're worried that he could injure the baby. What should we do?'

Respect starts at home

What's striking here? These parents only express concern about the new arrival, yet how do they themselves feel when their child hits them? By adopting the attitude that it 'doesn't bother us' we undermine our own self-esteem, and invite a child to go on behaving 'badly.'

Let's ask ourselves: what has this two-and-a-half-year-old child learned in his life so far that makes him treat his parents this way, as though they were some object like a table? The table says nothing when the child knocks against it because it's an inanimate object and cannot respond. Mum and Dad, on the other hand, are people. The way we allow ourselves to be treated has importance far beyond our own personal feelings. The child learns from his parents, the first and most important people in his life, that what he can do with Mum and Dad is OK, and that's how he will relate to others. The child will transfer this to other places and situations.

Avoid the Cinderella trap

Parents often hope that children will grow out of aggressive behaviour. This is a vain hope; the opposite is true.

The mother of a thirteen-year-old girl is in despair because her daughter, she says, 'drives her round the bend' with every little thing. 'Aren't there pills that can be prescribed for something like this?' she asks. 'People invent all sorts of things; they can even go to the moon. There must be a solution.'

There are no miracle pills for raising children. We have to create the miracles ourselves, and this begins with self-respect. This is the bottom line. Without it, you are pre-programmed for having difficulties in raising a child.

'For your humanity to be all-embracing and perfect, you must ... also have an attentive heart for yourself.'[3] The Bible likewise reminds us that a sense of our own dignity is important: 'Love thy neighbour as thyself.'

A sense of self-worth involves taking responsibility and being honest with oneself. We should feel that our own human dignity is violated if we tolerate attacks from a child without a word of objection. The child's acts of aggression are actually nothing other than cries for help.

So let's avoid the Cinderella trap of 'It doesn't bother me.' It does! Instead, do what's needed: be truthful and honest and say no, clearly, when a child oversteps her boundaries (see Chapter 1, p.18 for practical advice on how to do this). Give children the message that when you say no, you really mean it!

Clear boundaries

Clear boundaries are honest and necessary, and must be immediately drawn. By doing so, we no longer make it the child's 'fault' for being so difficult in daily life, but instead we adults take responsibility.

As parents we are not only entitled to bring up our children but obliged to do so. It is our duty to tell our child what is allowed and what is not — this is necessary even when there are other people around.

The German philosopher Novalis says that 'the human being learns humanity from human beings,' a vital piece of wisdom. Children need to be set examples by adults whom they can respect and who give them emotional security. Parents are in the front line here. When children lash out we should immediately put a stop to it and teach them not to do to others what you don't wish to be done to you.

Deal with conflict straight away

Translated into practice this means: 'Stop that, Simon! We do not have hitting here! And I'll tell you why: it hurts. I won't allow it.'

This follows all the rules of role clarity (see p.18). The same applies to other forms of assault: kicking, biting, spitting, scratching are all inappropriate, whoever it is directed at. If it happens, then assert the boundaries immediately: 'No! Stop that!' Insulting words are also inappropriate and the emergency brake should be applied: 'I won't allow this.' This works even when older children become abusive: 'Stop that, Becky. Don't speak to me like that. Please come back and talk to me when you've calmed down.'

Conflict is normal and children test us with it. It's wrong to avoid conflict as it just makes everything worse in the end. So don't be falsely 'good-natured,' don't ignore conflict or be vague in your response. Let's respond to conflict as a bull to a red rag. Rather than sweeping it under the carpet, place it squarely on the table, because all behaviour is learned. A child who is not taught what she can and cannot do will inevitably be hampered in her social behaviour and adjustment.

Respect for food

'No,' says Mum as Lawrence tries to take a second piece of cake. She points to his plate. 'Look, you've got a piece here that you've already started. Eat that one up first.' Lawrence still tries to take the new piece — as children do to see if adults really mean what they say. Of course they mean it, for otherwise all previous efforts would be wasted. In this instance, the mother gently takes the three-year-old's hand away from the big cake plate and repeats: 'Look, Lawrence, you've still got cake on your plate. Eat that one first.' And now Lawrence has understood.

What's striking here? In this family there is respect for food: Lawrence is not allowed more food as there is still food on his plate. This is teaching practical values: food is not taken arbitrarily and then thrown away afterwards because there was, after all, too much.

And why does Lawrence understand this relatively quickly? Instead of an irritated 'No, no, no, why can't you understand it?' going in one ear and out the other, this no is accompanied by an action. The mother gently but quite clearly takes the child's hand away from the big cake plate and points to the already bitten piece. This is a tangible, clear no, which the child can understand.

No, I don't allow that

Children don't initially have a sense of boundaries, but they endlessly try to find them, each day anew, even the youngest ones. Even small infants need very clear boundaries. Even if it doesn't hurt when your small child's fist lands in your face, you need to give a clear response, such as shaking your head or holding the child's hand and saying clearly, 'No, I don't allow that.'

What is important here, again, is to accompany the no with an action — a clear 'No' with a shake of your head to emphasize it, and take the child's hand away. Little children will understand this and once will be enough — here and now, in this particular situation.

Practising good habits

'But we already dealt with that this morning, and now we've got to go through it all over again. I can't keep telling you the same thing.' This would be fine if a child were to remember everything the first time, but for children once is nothing — just as they don't learn to stand at the first attempt but try again and again until they get the hang of it. This is why the 'good habits' we want to teach children have to be repeated many, many times. Skills are learned through repetition, and this gives children self-confidence.

Respect is giving and taking

We can also hold up a mirror to ourselves and — since we expect respect from them — look closely at how we speak to children. So often adults refer to them with expressions like 'Well, little tyrant ...' or 'you monster' or 'you little minx.'

A father said to his sons one evening, 'Well, you terrorists, what have you been up to today?' When asked why he addressed his sons like this, he replied, 'Oh, it's just a joke!' But from the child's point of view? Such expressions can be deeply wounding, even if they laugh at the time, out of uncertainty, because the grown-ups find it amusing. Let's not deceive ourselves: words are deeds. What has once been said can never be taken back. It has an effect. And that is why this saying from the Talmud is particularly relevant to child rearing.

> Attend to your thoughts, for they become words.
> Attend to your words, for they become deeds.
> Attend to your deeds, for they become habits.

Sensitivity to others

Respect is sensitivity to others — and no one is born with it. Respect makes life human and is learned only through example. Especially in the family, where people live in such close proximity to one another and each is aware of the other's weaknesses, showing respect on a daily basis is an important practice. Being respectful to your partner as much as to children and others simply means valuing another person, which has a wholesome effect. Those who feel valued learn to value themselves.

Our example is decisive. If I want something from someone then I should address them by name and make eye contact rather than saying, as it were in passing, 'Come on now, I've already told you ...' Giving one's full attention to the other person is one of the small gifts of respect.

Robert is all ears because he hears his name spoken. His mother looks at him. 'Robert, please help me lay the table.' The same to Sarah: 'Sarah, please tidy your shoes away.'

Say the child's name and then a brief request: this is neither stern nor old-fashioned but polite. Respect starts in small things, in daily life, and the more of it we give, the more peaceful we find our daily interactions.

Daily childcare relaxes as soon as we lead the way by good example. When we take care to speak to children with respect, the whole thing acquires a certain mood, and adults and children can grow together (see also Chapter 3, p.37).

I'm sorry

As parents we often only notice that we've treated our child disrespectfully after the event, like this father.

Today he's in a particular hurry, and today of all days — it seems to him — the little one is dawdling more than ever. The father explodes. He shouts furiously at his son and carries him downstairs to the car. Bad atmosphere — and also bad conscience. At the door of the kindergarten he suddenly feels guilty.

And now? Does he just leave it at that? Thankfully not. He does something exemplary. He bends down to his son and says, 'Ben, I'm really sorry that I shouted at you like that. Please forgive me; I didn't mean to.'

It is exemplary because the child learns something very decisive: that people make mistakes, and if they do then it is important to say sorry — to leap over one's own shadow, even if it's difficult. To ask for forgiveness is truly human and exemplary. It is balm for respectful interaction and develops the finest sensitivity for others.

The fundamental gestures of respect start with we adults: I respect myself; I respect you. This is the path from I to you in the world, and considerably reduces the stresses of raising children. 'True education,' as the proverb goes, 'is education of the heart.'

3. Rules

'I do make rules,' said a mother, 'but they are no use. My James never follows them.' James is four. The mother complains about tidying up. 'My son is perfectly aware that he has to tidy his things away in the evening, but at the most he chucks a couple of bricks in the box and then he just goes on playing as if I hadn't said anything.'

Why isn't it working with tidying up? Let's take a closer look. The mother describes what she does: 'Well, before supper, I tell my son, "It's time to tidy up please."' But what is the mother doing in the meantime? 'Mostly I'm cooking supper. And now and then I come out of the kitchen and check that he's getting on with it. Until I've had enough and then I get steamed-up and cross.'

This reminds me of the following story. A small crab is journeying with his mother. She keeps telling him off: 'For heaven's sake, walk straight. How many times do I have to tell you? Can't you hear me?' The little crab replies, 'Go ahead of me so I can see how to do it.'

Learning rules

'Go ahead of me.' This reply shows the golden bridge that children need for adhering to rules: 'Show me how.' It's like dancing: no one can learn it by words alone. We need someone to demonstrate how, repeatedly. For children the best way to acquire skills is to see how someone else does things and then do it too. This applies to tidying-up as well.

As parents, we are our children's first and most important teachers. Therefore we should show children what is right and encourage them to try it for themselves. 'Do it like the grown-ups.' Of course it takes a while to get established. Rome wasn't built in a day.

'Come on, let's do it together.'

This will certainly be necessary in the first four, five or six years of life — until it's become habit. Our example is decisive here. If you join in with the task yourself, the child will see how the desired task gets done quickly and happily.

But be careful, our own attitude is the important thing. If we undertake the necessary tasks, like tidying-up, unwillingly, children will notice and also reflect that. Children reflect every example that we give them back to us. Only one thing helps them to acquire a positive attitude to tasks: that we leave the daily grind behind for a moment and bring a fresh enjoyment to the activity.

These rules help

We need rules for potentially stressful situations, such as in the mornings, so that things run as smoothly as possible when everyone has to leave the house. We need rules to avoid evening chaos. We also need rules for mealtimes.

Rules save annoyance and exasperating confrontations. Tidying-up gets easier when there are clear rules to follow, which have been discussed beforehand and then demonstrated by example.

First rule

Tidying-up should always happen at the same time — preferably before supper. You can have a little transition ritual (see also 'Rhyme and sing-song' in Chapter 5, p.60).

But what to do if children haggle: 'Just a bit longer ...?'

Second rule

Be consistent. No negotiations or cajoling. Instead, say clearly and lovingly, 'Yes, James, I know you'd like to go on playing. But it's still time to tidy up. So we will.' This is important for children and gives them the experience that parents can't be swayed, but that what they say is reliable. This gives them security. We parents are the models for following rules.

My child has poor table manners

'My daughter always eats with her fingers. I'm tired of looking at it. We keep saying that she shouldn't, and that she shouldn't keep wiping her dirty fingers everywhere, but it does no good.'

The situation seems unresolvable. The child is in a role in which she experiences herself as powerful. And that is unhealthy, because by nature she needs something quite different.

According to Janusz Korczak, a great friend to children, 'The child wants to be taken seriously. He asks for trust, and expects guidance.'[4] Transposed to this theme of mealtimes, this means, firstly, the parents' trust: 'Yes, I trust that you can eat nicely.' And now for the guidance — but what and how?

What do we want to happen?

Let's first consider what needs to change. What do we want to happen at mealtimes? An important rule might be, 'In our house we use cutlery to eat.' From what age should such rules apply? Start as early as possible. A spoon is fine from six months and a fork from about the age of one. Of course food will go astray to begin with, but practice makes perfect and children are proud when they master a skill.

Be consistent

This applies, too, to rules for mealtimes: 'In our house we use cutlery to eat.' No discussion. It is a rule that is followed. Being consistent is an important aid to stress-free parenting. Parents' uncertainty, on the other hand, makes everything more complicated, such as here: 'Sometimes,' says a mother, 'my son allows himself to be persuaded to use a spoon or fork, but this is rare. That's why we mostly have food that he can eat with his hands, such as noodles, carrots, beans, fish fingers and bread.'

What's wrong with that? It's the sense of partnership, the need to 'persuade' and then the caving in: 'Oh, you'd prefer to eat with your fingers — OK then.' The child finds himself in a position of power with the result that mealtimes become stressful times and equanimity flies out of the window.

Discussing rules in advance

It's best to try to implement new rules when tempers aren't frayed. Rules must always be discussed beforehand. In the case of mealtimes, this would mean not stating rules when things have become stressed during the meal, but beforehand, while everyone is still relaxed.

And what if it doesn't work? Of course, we learn on the job. This always means repeatedly practising and learning clarity of roles. Recalling the five rules from page 18, this means:

1. Not discussing things by-the-by but with complete attention.
2. Saying the child's name so that he understands it is really him who is meant.
3. Making eye contact. The human gaze touches the child inwardly and he feels addressed.
4. Saying clearly what you want: 'In our house we use cutlery to eat. From today you can do this too.' Then remind him once, shortly before the meal, and show trust: 'You'll be able to do this.' When a child sees trust in the adult's eyes this encourages him more than a thousand promptings. If the child still uses his fingers nevertheless, it's time for the next rule.
5. Keep your eye on the ball and make sure that these rules are really followed. This makes us adults predictable in a child's eyes. And you can use a touch of humour: 'Remember our rules, Julia? They're for everyone — you too! Ok, let's try again.'

Social rules for daily life

Daily life improves considerably if we follow a few social rules: we say hello when we come home; we put our hand in front of our mouth when we yawn; we blow our nose in a handkerchief; we put rubbish in the bin; when something falls down we pick it up straight away; no mobile calls at mealtimes. Naturally such rules must apply to everyone, and they have to be established, because what is not learned by the child does not develop into a skill (see also Chapter 9, p. 95).

If rules are ignored

Now things get interesting. We adults must maintain, clearly and precisely, that the rule holds good, rather than becoming uncertain. This is important. Why? Children must learn that there are things that must be done, for example, taking out the rubbish. And this will happen if we persevere: 'That's what's going to happen now. Please take the rubbish out. No discussion.'

I don't want to be strict

Many parents are worried about being too strict and potentially losing their children's affection. But this fear is unfounded. Being clear means giving the child security. This is different from bring strict. Strictness, in contrast, involves the 'consequences principle' such as saying, 'If you don't clean your teeth now, there'll be no story.'

Parents often do this and feel bad about it afterwards. We can avoid this if we say clearly, 'This is what's happening. We're doing this now ...' and then apply the known rule.

Of course it's always uncomfortable to keep insisting. But there's no alternative, for our children's sake. Our clarity tells them where they are, and they long for this: here is someone who knows what's what, who knows what should happen and does not spin in every breeze like a weather vane.

'And if my child shouts?' He may. No cause for worry. Children like to test whether a rule is watertight. Of course it is! Otherwise all your efforts will come to nothing.

Repetition of sequences

Rules help you when daily life has become stressful. Daily activities like arriving home belong here. It can run smoothly if everything always follows the same sequence: taking coats off straight away and hanging on a hook in the corridor; placing outdoor shoes in the same place each time then putting on slippers; then washing your hands. Everything happens each time in the same sequence. This isn't pedantic but creates order and the right conditions for them to learn and act independently.

Getting up, washing, dressing, eating, brushing teeth or tidying up — everything goes more smoothly if it's always done in a regular sequence. For example, if a child is about to get dressed:

* Always get dressed in the same place, for instance next to the same stool in the child's bedroom.
* Put the clothes on in the same order, for instance, first pants, then T-shirt, then socks, then jumper and finally trousers.

The same principle applies for everything. Children learn by *doing*. 'Regular' means that what happens today will happen tomorrow, the next day, in a week, in a month ...

Repetition helps to establish and internalize what needs to be done. It becomes a sustaining habit and saves tedious arguments and exhortations; and children no longer have to test everything endlessly.

Media rules

Clear rules are also essential for watching television, playing video games and Internet use. Young children shouldn't be in front of the television: the screen is not a harmless window on the world. Sitting in front of it tempts them to spend more and more time doing the same — with harmful consequences, as scientific research has shown.[5] Image media has become our new child-raising partner of the 21st century, and increasingly this assumes an addictive character, leading children to develop a brain that can adapt to virtual reality but not to real life.

Setting rules is the number one piece of advice for parents. Let's sit down with them and see for a moment what children are exposed to: 'What a load of garbage' said a father, who followed this advice. After this he found it very easy to establish firm rules for viewing times: what, when and how long. And enforcing this? 'It works OK, just as with other necessary rules: the more sure I am myself, the less protest there is.'

Another positive side effect: 'Since I've been setting clear rules,' says a mother of teenagers, 'my children respect me again. Although they are often annoyed, I think they notice that I'm not concerned with power, with laying down the law, but with them as people.'

It doesn't always have to be heavy

It isn't always necessary to come down like a ton of bricks if a rule is not followed. A lighter touch is often better.

Sebastian's dirty shoes are lying in the middle of the corridor. His father remarks with a smile, 'Do you want us to admire your shoes by leaving them in the middle of the floor?' Or to Florian, who comes to a meal without washing his hands, 'Oops, I think someone's forgotten to wash their hands.'

The effect is astonishing. A remark like that is like a little reminder. The child was testing whether the rule was really watertight or not. Now he knows he has been seen, and feels, 'Ah, I really am important to you!' A smile, and the child is motivated to do the task, and everyone can relax.

4. Rhythm

It's nearly 11 p.m. and Oscar is still rushing about. He's four years old and has been making himself the centre of attention all evening. His drinking glass has just slipped out of his hand and the tablecloth is now covered with juice.

'Right, that's enough now!' his mother calls out, annoyed, and decisively takes her son to bed.

When she returns to her invited guests shortly afterwards, one of them says, 'Well, you could have done that three hours ago ...'

'Hardly,' she replies, 'he's been a nuisance all evening, saying that he isn't tired yet.'

Randomness is unsettling

How easy it is to tell a child, 'You're being a nuisance!' But in this situation it isn't just the adults who are on edge. The child is as well. More than that, he's very stressed. And why? Once again it's this 'partnership' behaviour: 'Do you want to? Ah, you don't want to yet, OK ... What would you like to do?' It is simply asking too much of children to treat them like equal partners. This continual asking and trying to please always leads to conflict (see Chapter 1, p. 13).

If we as parents prefer to be our child's friend rather than bring her up, everything gets difficult: evening bedtimes, mealtimes and very often the beginning of the day. A father once told me, 'My son is four. He's a lovely boy but every morning he drives me up the wall.'

Here we have this 'being on edge' again. And then children are often blamed, though often wrongly. If the sequence of the day is chaotic, without firm habits, children will be stressed. Stressed children pass on their stress, stressing those around them. And this eats away at the whole family's life forces — until people lose their joy in their children and everyone feels exhausted.

The miracle of rhythm

Nature itself, and our own bodies, are exemplary, showing how the smallest to the most complex processes and sequences can function smoothly. Just think of the heartbeat or breathing that keep us alive. How does all this work without great fuss and bother? The miracle is called rhythm and always follows the same principle. A process occurs:

* at a particular location
* in a particular way
* at a particular interval of time

Pause and *repetition:* the same thing recurs repeatedly — at the same location, in the same way, and at the same interval. Regular. Reliable.

All life functions like this, starting from the smallest cell to the big rhythms of the planets: day — night; day — night. The underlying principle of rhythm is reliable repetition.

'Repetition,' according to the researcher Anne Jean Ayres, saves 'nervous energy'.[6] And this is exactly what we need for raising children. Translated into everyday family life this means that having regular sequences that occur at particular times will save us and our children distress, annoyance and edgy discussions.

A clear rhythm to the day

How can we incorporate a helpful rhythm into daily family life? The best thing is to be very practical: sit down with a paper and pencil and in one column first write down the major recurring events of every day. For instance, the children Clara and James have the same sequence each morning:

* they are woken
* they get up
* they go to the bathroom
* they get dressed
* they have breakfast together with the family
* they go to the bathroom again
* they put on their shoes and coat
* they leave the house to go to kindergarten and school

Put the actual times at which these events happen alongside the list.

'Does it have to be so exact? Is that really necessary?' Yes, to begin with definitely, because then we as parents gain the clarity we need.

In the same way as for the morning we need regular times in the family for eating, homework, play, going out, practising musical instruments and relaxing in the evening.

We can involve the children in this if we write down what happens each day in clear writing on a large sheet of paper, and encourage them to draw or paint little pictures to illustrate it. For instance, a sun next to the time for waking up, a toothbrush for brushing teeth ... You can pin up the sheet in a visible place such as a kitchen door or a pinboard in the corridor. Then we will see it all the time as we pass by, and this will encourage us to really implement it.

Always the same place

Dressing, homework and eating are always best done in the same place. This makes things clearer. Children have a good 'location memory' but not yet a strategy for learning. This is why they are so dependent on our clear guidance.

On home visits and in consultations I have found that many families no longer even have a dining table. But this is essential. The dining table is a power place, important for the whole family. Everyone — and especially children — need regular meals that are eaten at this particular place, both in the morning and evening. If children are at home then at lunchtime too. Meals should not happen alongside other things: they are a cultural, social and health-enhancing event. The first thing I recommend to families without a dining table is to go out and buy one!

Day–night rhythm

Our children gain strength from a reliable day–night rhythm. To introduce this with the necessary assurance, it's good if we know exactly how much sleep a child needs at each age. An infant of three months needs between thirteen and fifteen hours of sleep, split into about five hours during the day and the rest of at night, waking up once or twice in the night. Kindergarten-age children still need about twelve hours of sleep, school children around ten to eleven hours. 'Oh, my child isn't getting nearly enough then,' say many parents when they hear this.

Why is adequate sleep so important?

Good sleep is important so that children can develop well in all ways. Forces used up during the day are regenerated in sleep. The breathing rhythm levels off and the day's experiences are 'digested.' The child's organs, including the brain, grow during sleep. For children to get enough sleep at night, they need relatively strict bedtimes. Going to bed can become a highpoint of the day with lovely little rituals (see Chapter 5, p.63).

Night is night

Sleeping at night has to be practised. Waking up at night is quite normal for infants, but it is easier to reduce this as soon as possible if we adults make the minimum fuss about it — for instance, the least amount of light. Use calming gestures of care and comfort. On no account start playing, cuddling, dandling or activities that might make waking up at night an interesting prospect.

Practising rhythm

Once a helpful daily rhythm has been established, it has to be practised. These things don't happen from one day to the next; it's a journey that gets easier each time the same sequences recur. This relieves everyone, because everyone knows where they stand.

Introducing new, helpful rhythms takes at least a month. And there is only one way to do it: repetition. As highlighted, the principle underlying rhythm is that a process recurs at a particular interval. It is repeated reliably — at the same place and in the same way.

There is power in repetition! Eventually, one day, situations that were once stressful will no longer be so.

Enjoying rhythm in daily life

Rhythm is enhanced and enlivened by recurring rituals (see Chapter 5). It will then no longer feel like a merely schematic thing, like a school timetable, but will acquire qualities that invoke joyful action and feeling in the child. Repeating rhythms that recur in the same way each day gives a child the sense that things will be like this today, tomorrow and the next day, and therefore she feels secure and safe. This is painfully lacking when we — supposedly liberally — say, 'Let her decide herself when she wants to eat.' Children don't yet have a clear idea of their real needs. A well-known German magazine recently ran a cover article entitled 'Come on, bring me up please!'[7]

Rhythm makes it easier to bring children up. There is much less argument, annoyance and irritation. You don't have to keep negotiating, discussing or battling your way through shouting and crying because children can rely on what is already familiar. This gives them security.

5. Rituals

The father taps on the five fingertips of his son's small hand. 'Five more sleeps and then it will be your birthday.'

'Oh ... yes. Will we go to the big meadow again? Are we going to play those fun games again?'

Children are masters of ceremony. They want what happened last time to happen in the same way next time, without change. In this sense children are very old-fashioned: they really don't want new occurrences all the time. They want rituals — not just on special days such as their birthday, Christmas, Easter and other festive days, but every day.

Are we going to do it again?

If we're attentive, we find that children have a sense of what is good for them and gives them a sense of security: 'Are we going to do it again?' The shared experience is important: the adult who repeats a ritual with them belongs intrinsically to it.

To do something again in the same way as before is taxing for parents today, since repeating something we already know is completely at odds with modern life. But it's worth adapting and taking the child's deep need for stability seriously. Where something positive is repeated each time in the same way, we are no longer acting against the child's nature but in harmony with it. Harmonizing rituals are important anchors in stress-free parenting. They considerably ease family life.

Rituals ease transition

In everyday family life, one situation changes frequently into another. Change is always associated with uncertainty, and that's when things are likely to get difficult, for example, at the transition from play to tidying-up (see also Chapter 3, p.37). Rituals help to mark and ease potentially tricky situations, and also enliven and animate them.

Momentary blossoms

Rituals, whether elaborate or simple, always address the feelings. They are like momentary blossoms that we adults can bring to flower. There are many opportunities for this in daily family life.

Lisa has fallen over and is crying pitifully. The next moment it's
all over. She sniffs a couple of times and then a smile passes across
her face.

What was so effective? A little healing rhyme.

Here's a little blessing:
First three days of pouring rain
Then three days of shining sun
And soon all will be well again.

These parents only recently discovered this. 'Before,' they said,
'we always talked and asked much too much: "Where's it hurting?
Why didn't you watch where you were going?" and so on. This
just made Lisa cry even louder, and it took ages to calm her down
again.'

Such partner-like discussion is, indeed, unhelpful. Continual
questioning requires children to say something reasonable back,
in the middle of their fright or hurt. But often all that is needed is
to be seen, touched and comforted. A little rhyme helps more than
all interrogation, for it always also addresses and soothes feelings.

Rituals with rhyme and song

'If they do not sing it, they will not believe it,' said Martin Luther
— a wonderful piece of wisdom, which is very helpful in daily life
with children. A rhyme or little song makes potentially stressful
transitions easier, for instance a song before tidying-up or washing
hands. The moment children hear a little melody in our voice,
they listen, which they often don't do if an order is simply given:
'Now wash your hands, I've told you already.' A rhyme is worth a
thousand words:

It's almost suppertime again —
Let's wash hands to get them clean.

This reaches children's hearts, and then they'll be on board. Of course, we wash our hands too, as an example!

The morning is golden

Starting the morning in a positive frame of mind colours the rest of the day. A loving good-morning ritual awakens positive feelings and creates a good mood, making both adults and children feel happy.

A ritual expressing the fact that 'I'm pleased to see you' can involve a loving touch such as a good morning kiss, stroking and cuddling. Rituals are always individual, so we should choose whatever best suits us personally.

Oh, I see, it's me they're talking to

It's important to be called by one's own name right at the start of the day. All of us, not just children, grow a little more awake and attentive when we hear our own name spoken. 'Oh, I see, it's me they're talking to ...' A simple rhyme that accompanies this is uplifting for a child:

Good morning my Peter
Good morning I say
Good morning dear Peter
It's a lovely new day.

A morning prayer can also be enlivening if this is something you have an authentic relationship with (see Chapter 10, p.105).

These first moments of the day can give a child an enjoyable, peaceful sense of being cared for, being really 'parented' and this helps them get out of bed on the right side. It's quite different from just saying, 'Time to get up, the bathroom's free!'

Greetings and goodbyes

Greetings and goodbyes are part of the core rituals in family life. These are moments when we can really perceive each other for a moment. It's important to look the child in the eye at such times.

Why isn't it enough just to say hello in passing or a hip 'hey' to a teenager? Greeting and goodbye rituals offer brief moments of togetherness, a sense of you and me; they can repeatedly be a touchstone for nurturing a relationship. This involves taking time, even if just a couple of seconds: I look at you. I see you. I'm pleased. I greet you. These are small sources of strength that do everyone in the family good. We all need them regularly.

And how do Mum and Dad greet each other when one of them comes home? Our behaviour is an example to children, and forms them. So it's not just a matter of doing everything right for the child but also, as a couple, of exchanging some loving greeting and goodbye rituals. The child learns socially desirable behaviour from this.

Physical contact and nest warmth

Loving physical contact is part of many little family rituals: embracing and a kiss when saying hello and goodbye, and at other moments. This is like an elixir, and children need it at least three times a day. Every contact with the skin, our largest sensory organ, addresses the whole person. These rituals give security and self-confidence, establishing a sense of 'we.' This is a sustaining element that creates the whole family's identity.

Rituals involving physical contact are needed when a child wakes up, when he goes out of the house, at bedtime (see also Chapter 9, p.102), and to comfort him; also, of course, when crossing the road and in other unpredictable situations.

A ritual involving physical contact is also helpful for beginning a meal together peacefully: holding hands for a moment, making eye contact and maybe even a simple grace, either spoken or sung. Little rituals like this give a quiet pause in the often busy day. Being touched touches children inwardly (see Chapter 9, p.100).

Ending the day in tranquility

When the day ends and children are ready for bed — always at the same time (see Chapter 4, p.50) — a lovely goodnight ritual is a gift to them. It's important to have the same sequence each night: a story and, if you feel comfortable with this, an evening prayer — or whatever feels right for you. To end, as prelude to sleep, the same farewell ritual, personal to you and the child. No machine, TV or music player can replace what Mum or Dad can give. You can sing a good-night song together, for instance; it doesn't have to be perfectly performed or even perfectly in tune. The crucial thing is that *you* sing it, as well as you can manage. The following poem by William Blake has a lovely, peaceful quality. You could make up a simple tune to go with it.

From *Night*

The sun descending in the west,
The evening star does shine;
The birds are silent in their nest,
And I must seek for mine.

The moon like a flower
In heaven's high bower,
With silent delight
Sits and smiles on the night.

Farewell green fields and happy groves
Where flocks have took delight.
Where lambs have nibbled, silent moves
The feet of angels bright.
Unseen they pour blessing
And joy without ceasing
On each bud and blossom
And each sleeping bosom.

And after these or other calming words, which enfold a child in a sense of security, a good-night kiss and good wishes for sweet dreams.

6. Responsiveness

'These infants are to be provided only with the barest essentials: food, suckling and clothing. No one may speak to them, smile at them or embrace them.' This, according to Horst Eberhard in his book about Frederick Barbarossa,[8] *was ordered by the latter in an experiment designed to discover the archetypal human language. Newborn babies were brought together in a room where their nurses followed these instructions to the letter. The experiment came to a dramatic end after a few weeks: as Eberhard describes it, the infants 'were no longer able to live without the touch, friendly looks and words of endearment from their nurses.'*

What was lacking was the primary quality we all need in order to connect with the world: the live-giving mutuality of responsiveness — for only by meeting a 'you' can the 'I' awaken.

First smiles

At around four to six weeks a child smiles for the first time, at first unconsciously. This has been called the 'angel smile.' Only through a response from parents does the 'smile dialogue' develop. Encouraged by the joy reflected in her parents' faces, she smiles again. Smiling and being smiled at, giving and taking — responsiveness. Children need loving interaction, gestures, touch and above all eye contact.

To be seen is *the* great need of children. A poem by Hilde Domin runs:[9]

> *You are*
> *because eyes want you,*
> *look at you and say*
> *that you are.*

This inner attention is existentially necessary for the child: 'The parents' perceiving smiles protect the child against negative stress that she is exposed to as she develops ... She responds less anxiously or aggressively as long as this dialogue of smiles, in which she feels perceived, is a sufficiently frequent experience.'[10]

Is the child thriving?

You can see in a child's eyes whether she is thriving. Children's eyes shine when we are responsive to them, and they gain this little pleasure in a very simple way through finding games. Little ones just hide their eyes: 'Look — where am I?' Slightly older ones hide under a table or behind the curtain — first a brief moment of suspense, and then radiant looks when the adult finds them:

'Here I am!' It's wonderful, this feeling of being looked for, being important: 'Mum or Dad is pleased to find me and see me.'

Little response games

If the child is happy the parents are happy, and vice versa. If things get a bit stressful with children, it's a good idea to leave everything else to one side for a moment and play games with eye contact: hide-and-seek, cuddling games, hand and finger games. Just a couple of minutes of this will work miracles. Little response games are a real source of strength and always end in warm laughter. Laughter lifts and liberates the spirits and is infectious; pleasure gives new strength. According to St Augustine, 'Pleasure nourishes the soul.'

Response blockers

Children need a great deal of response, also in order to learn to speak. They need to be spoken to a lot, since learning to speak only comes from speaking. This sounds obvious, but it's important to be fully aware of it, and to practise it — as shown by the dramatic increase in children suffering from speech development disorders. Parents are seeking advice in ever greater numbers because their child has not yet started to speak at sixteen or seventeen months, or even by the age of two, but instead still just babbles.

Being more aware of the effect of fashionable 'response blockers' will do a lot to remedy this problem. These include buggies that do not allow the child and parent to see each other, and also dummies (pacifiers) and pacifier bottles, or continually offering a child things to munch on when out and about.

Children have only recently arrived in the world, and they learn everything by becoming accustomed to it. If they continually have something in their mouths they can learn to suppress their natural impetus to speak, and will then consider this normal.

Response blockers waste precious opportunities for conversation. Learning to speak develops in the most natural and best way if we speak to the child from birth in proper speech, and talk *with* her as much as possible when she's awake. Although children may hear speech on the radio or television, this is meaningless to them because it has no relationship context that really includes them. Research has shown that delayed speech development is often connected with early exposure to these media.[11]

Enjoying responsiveness

A father has just arrived at the bus stop with his small son. He turns the buggy round to face him and talks to the little boy. Now he's puffing up his cheeks and blowing raspberries, and then repeats this. The one-year-old beams, his whole body expressing pleasure through to his fingertips and toes. 'We do this every morning,' says the father. He's taking the boy to the childminder. 'I use our journey to chat a bit. I really enjoy it,' he says, 'and it strengthens my sense of being a dad.'

What's happening when a child cries?

Often we reach without thinking for a dummy or pacifier if a child starts crying. 'What else can I do? I can't just let my child cry ...'

True enough but, as Alice Miller highlights so emphatically, it's important to let children articulate their anger and pain without feeling at risk of losing their parents' love and care.[12] Even when a child is hysterical, responsiveness helps.

A family is on the train. Their infant is crying. His mother leans over him and looks at him warmly. She lays her hand on his tummy and leaves it there: 'Yes, darling Leon, you're crying, aren't you? Tell me what the matter is; I'm listening. Mm, I can't understand what's wrong at the moment. But I'm here ...' She keeps her hand there and stays turned towards the child.

It is magical to witness this. The child sobs a couple of times more but in a couple of minutes his distress has been soothed.

Telling and healing

What is so valuable about this interaction? It's the invitation to say what's wrong. Telling almost has the word 'healing' concealed in it. Healing occurs the moment the child's energy isn't suppressed. No dummy, bottle or other pacifier, but responsiveness. The mother turns her full attention to her child. She maintains eye contact, uses endearments and speaks his name, touching his tummy and keeping her hand in contact there. 'Yes, I'm listening, darling, tell me even if I can't understand at the moment.' It's effective, astonishingly quickly.

According to the latest research, so-called reflective neurons are at work here.[13] Even very young children actually respond to what others think and feel.

And with older children?

Every child is on a quest for acknowledgment, esteem and a sense of belonging, for contact and response; and first and foremost she wants this from her parents.

All children at every age need responsiveness, particularly

when something's gone wrong — for instance with friends at school, or because a best friend is moving away. Your relationship with your child will benefit simply from you placing your hand on hers and trying to sense how she's feeling right now.

Gestures are often more important than lots of words. Instead of firing off questions, therefore, just try focusing completely on your child. That's love, which is more than words.

Feeling resonance

Resonance and responsiveness have a healing effect, also at bedtime. Did we perceive our child enough today? Did we listen to her properly? After the busy, perhaps hectic day, do we know how our child is feeling?

As parents it's important to develop a sense for this. Children have often had an enormously taxing day — in a big group with many others in nursery, at kindergarten or school. Often they have to cope with far more each day than we realize.

Quality time

Quality time brings parents and children back together again. In the evening, at a particular time, you can settle down in a nice chair and perhaps light a candle: 'Now I'm completely here for you.' You can put the child on your lap and hold her securely, and simply sit there in silence, just listening and sensing. Undivided attention — three minutes is enough.

If we manage to open our ears and heart completely for this brief period, a small miracle will happen every evening: the child calms down. Her breathing grows noticeably calmer, the tension passes from her limbs. She feels that someone is there who really has time for her, who wants to hear what she says. And usually she will begin to tell you something — often something that's bothering her.

Such a clear sign of attention and responsiveness answers the child's deep longing: 'I am simply acknowledged as I am.'

7. Reassurance

A king and queen had all they could wish for — except a child. At last, as the Grimms' fairy tale relates, God granted their wish. But when the child was born he did not look like a human child but like a young donkey ...

His father, however, continued to support his son: 'God gave him to us, and he will remain my son and heir.' The young donkey, as the tale says, learned many skills, including playing the lyre. And thus he succeeded in winning the love of a beautiful princess and could lay aside his donkey form for ever.

'All things are possible ...'

'... to him who believes,' the Bible says. This king gave his son the most precious thing that parents can give a child — he believed in him unconditionally: 'You don't have to be what I expect or imagine, but I will do everything to ensure that you can fulfil your potential.' Such reassurance and loving support opens worlds. The child can reveal his potential, what he bears within him.

Children want to show what they can do

Children want to show their innate capacities, and are happy to exert themselves — even the youngest — when they're learning to stand and walk. Soon after they will insist, 'On my own!' Little ones want to eat with their spoon, put on their own socks and much more. What children need here is reassurance and loving support: 'You can start and I'll help a little if you need it.' It's important to help a child to make his own efforts. Don't worry if it takes a long time, but enjoy the fact that children become increasingly independent.

So often parents ask, 'How can I nurture my child?' In the endless wealth of programmes and courses on parenting, we should not overlook the need to reinforce children's skills in daily life, which we as parents are primarily responsible for.

Trust works miracles

Sometimes children look for the easy option.

A seven-year-old has to draw a tree for homework: 'I can't draw a tree,
can you do one for me?'
      'Just draw it however you like!'
      But the child insists: 'I can't do it!'
      'Just try.'
      Keep insisting. Trusting instead of rushing to help will encourage
tentative children.
      A couple of minutes later, he calls out a happy, 'Look what I did!'
He was able to draw a tree after all.

What does the child gain from this? He learns that he can help
himself and that this strengthens his sense of self-esteem.

But what if my child is being a nuisance?

'What an afternoon it's been,' complains a mother. 'Three times in
a row I had to wipe up apple juice from the kitchen floor. I've really
had enough now.'

What happens when we adults immediately clear up the mess
our children make? It gets done quicker. And what does the
child learn? That 'it doesn't matter what I do. It's nothing to
do with me.'

To engage fully with life, children absolutely need to learn to
clear up the mess they've made. This has to be practised from a
young age. Children need guidance in this and reassurance.

Let's do it together

In order to guide the child fully, go through the process with
them step by step: fetch a bucket with the child, fill it with
water, add cleaner, fetch a cloth. The child also gets one. Dip

the cloth in, then show how you wring it out well and wipe the floor with it. Take note of the child's efforts. What's important is to finish the cleaning together. 'And next time watch out a bit more, Jamie.' Perhaps you'll also see that Jamie suddenly grows a little inwardly, as he looks happily at what you've done together. He has just discovered that he can make something better again. And now you can take pleasure together in the good outcome: 'Look, how nice and tidy everything is again.' A little acknowledgment really helps.

No stress!

Children are children — sometimes they intentionally do something wrong.

Instead of showing his parents, Julian signed his mother's name to a reprimand he received from school. This came to light when his parents attended parents' evening. They talked to their son about it, saying why this was wrong, and how they felt: 'This wasn't right. We're sad about it because it's important to us that we're honest with each other.' The father said, 'It's not just that you forged the signature, Julian. What you did was bad, but you're not. We love you.'

The reassurance offered here is that they do not confuse the mischief with the child. This is vital. Many parents rightly want their children to trust them. This means children must be able to tell their parents about their worries without anxiety. It's possible that Julian was afraid of his parents' reactions to his school misdemeanour, and the forged signature was due to this.

When children don't do their chores

And now we come to the age-old story of the guinea pig, rabbit or hamster. The child longs for a little furry animal. At last the parents agree: 'But only if you clean his hutch out.' Of course he will!

The first two or three times he does so, but then enthusiasm wanes.

'I have to go on at him all the time,' complains a parent. 'There's always an argument about it.' What should I do?

There's no need for battles; the moment it's time to clean the hutch again, give loving support and simply remind him, 'Sam, it's time to clean the hutch.' Say it with conviction and certainty, not with the expectation of a showdown. Often a short, friendly, reminder will be enough.

The same applies to shoes left in the corridor, or unwashed hands. We should try reminding children before getting hot under the collar and launching into an argument.

Homework

A common complaint from parents is, 'It's so hard with my son. He can't focus properly on his homework. It's the same thing every day.' How can we offer reassurance and support here?

First consider whether he had a break after school to recoup his strength and energy. Loving support also means giving children guidance about how they can refresh themselves. Depending on temperament, he may need a rest (see Chapter 9, p.101), while another prefers to paint or draw (see Chapter 8, p.92). For yet another child, movement is the best thing after sitting still in school and on the bus, so out into the garden or the park for a runabout, or play on the swings or climbing frame.

After this break and renewal of energies, homework can begin. Homework time needs a fixed rhythm (see Chapter 4, p.50). It's very important that homework should be finished before the evening meal. Children need their relaxation time just like anyone else.

Simply being there

Jonathan had a tough exam today. The parents show interest: 'How did it go?'
'Oh, leave me alone.' He disappears into his room ...

The parents would like to help, but how? First let him calm down. Reassurance and support can be given later, when the anger's faded. There's one important thing to remember. If a child is having problems, don't ask, 'What can I do?' but think of something suitable and then do it. Two or three hours later, for instance, something like this is possible: 'I've made us a nice cup of hot chocolate. I'd like to sit down with you for a moment.'

There's no need to expect anything in particular. Don't try to get him to talk. Don't diminish what he's feeling by saying, 'I'm sure it's not so bad.' What's needed here is really to be present. 'I'm here if you want to talk to me — and if not, that's fine too.'

If the child does say what's wrong, then the most important thing is to listen. Listening doesn't yet solve the problem, but it eases the trouble, and the child will feel that there's a safe harbour where he can take refuge — however he's feeling.

Adding a supportive question can help a child to pick himself up: 'What do you think might help to make sure it goes better next time?'

Our teenagers still need this kind of loving support, however coolly they seem to signal that they can do without us. Deep in their hearts — particularly in difficult situations — they want their parents' support, for then they feel that their parents care about them, are not indifferent to them and still value them.

8. Room

In the middle of town. A father is pushing his four-year-old in a buggy through the pedestrian precinct; the mother is following, a sandwich in one hand and a colourful drinking bottle in the other, with a teat. 'Wait a moment!' she calls out. Now she offers the child the sandwich and bottle and asks, 'Would you like something?' An everyday city picture ...

Children need room to grow

Do adults act in this way because they want an easy life, to keep the child quiet? Offering her something to eat at every opportunity may be well-intentioned, and likewise, not asking anything of her, pushing or carrying her even though she has long been able to walk. But, whatever the reason, it comes at far too much of a cost.

When no demands are made of children, they lack the space to develop in a healthy way. This is demonstrated dramatically in current school entry tests. Doctors diagnose massive developmental disorders in every third to fourth child — such as impaired movement coordination, attention deficit and speech development disorders.

Interest

What can one do to avoid impaired development? As the saying goes, 'Children aren't a pot to be filled but a fire to be lit.' The fire is the wonderful energy of interest that every child brings with her into the world. By nature every child is eager to learn. She wants to be active, to move. She wants to discover things and experiment.

Children need space for their own autonomous activity to avoid their innate interest waning. They need space to find out things for themselves. We adults are examples to them in this. Everything we do or don't do in their presence is formative for them. Irrespective of whether something has a purpose and aim, they imitate us.

A mother gets out of the car with her two-year-old, and her mobile phone falls on the ground. The little girl bends down to get it. The mother is pleased at the thought of her returning it to her, but after fishing it out of the gutter she throws it onto the road with gusto. She's just seen her mother doing this, so she wants to do it too. Her reason is still dreaming; only the actions she witnesses awaken her interest and are imitated.

Imitation

Children learn to stand and walk through imitation. If things go well, this is how they acquire skills of all kinds. We can motivate children to develop their own capacities by giving them the space to do a task alongside us, *not* by sending them away because we can do it quicker without them (see also Chapter 1, p.17).

Cooking, baking and various kinds of work or repairs in the house and garden stimulate imitation.

Sarah is seven. She sees her mother sewing. 'I want to do that too!' She wants to 'sew something proper.' She's pleased at the idea of sewing the missing button back on to Dad's pyjamas. She threads the needle and sews, and her mother shows her how to finish it off at the end. The whole afternoon Sarah asks, 'When's Dad coming?' And how her eyes shine when he sees her little surprise — a light from within.

We can often see this inner glow; it lights up whenever children are engaged and interested in something, and are allowed to make or do something themselves.

Space for my own experiences

There's an old saying, 'Give me a rod, not a fish on a plate.' That's what children need, essentially: space to do things themselves, to discover things for themselves, to be allowed to do things. We can give them this space in everyday life.

To begin with, little children are very keen to 'join in.' As long as they are not spoiled by mollycoddling, tasks remain very interesting to them. Why? Because the grown-up does them; because children wish to be around the grown-up and do the same. That's why it's so important not to prevent them from joining in. Every time you say something like, 'Leave it now, I'll do it myself quickly,' children lose a little more of their enjoyment in being active themselves and acquiring skills. It's then hardly surprising then if, at some later point, they no longer have any inclination to do anything, like this eleven-year-old: her mother asks her to water the flowerbeds with the garden hose. Finally she does so with a sulky expression. Her mother says, 'If you don't want to, just leave it then.'

Why is this response so disastrous? Children do not engage with life if we remove every hindrance and only ask them to do what they 'want to.' They will then often show forms of behaviour which adults call 'difficult.'

Difficult?

A fax comes through: a photocopied newspaper article sent to a friend, and below it in handwriting the words, 'Read this article: it shows why our James is always so difficult. I'm sure he has ADHD as described here.'

The answer, by return of fax, runs: 'When was the last time you took your son for a walk in the wood? When did you last go for a whole day's hike with him, so that he was really tired in the evening and collapsed into bed? When did you set off together for an adventure, gather wood, build a fire in the open air or a dam in a river? Don't take offence — you know I mean well.'

Well meant, indeed, and also very practical.

In his book about the inhospitable nature of cities,[14] Alexander

Mitscherlich wrote that:

> The young person needs elemental things: water, muck,
> bushes, space to play. One can also let him grow up
> without all that, with carpets, soft animals or on asphalt
> streets and yards instead. He will survive — but it's not
> so surprising, later, if he has not acquired certain basic
> social capacities.

Children need space to play because, as Schiller said, 'The
human being is born free, free!' and is full of potential and innate
ability. It's life-enhancing for a child to play in a free and self-
determining way, following his own dictates and imagination.

Room for self-expression

Children need room to unfold their own forms of expression,
room for self-initiated games, and for movement, music, painting,
drawing or modelling. Why is this 'free space' so important?
Children take pleasure in their own activity, ability and creativity.
They draw life forces from such activity and strengthen their sense
of self-worth.

If we ask where, in our busy, modern lives, the child has such
space to pursue her own creativity, it becomes clear that children's
daily timetables need something different from what we adults
often regard as convenient.

They should include fixed times for play. Let's ensure this is
possible, every day. Children who play freely and devise their own
games acquire important skills for life — though not in any kind
of goal-oriented way — which stand them in good stead as adults:
'Children who learn to organize their own play cope better with
school work later on and become better-adjusted adults.'[15]

In addition, children benefit from being encouraged to paint and draw freely, rather than being presented with pre-printed painting templates. Free painting gives them a sense of their own vitality. If a child, such as five-year-old Martina, is used to pre-drawn schemas and does not dare paint without them, we could say, 'Imagine you're a rainbow. What would you look like?' A little guidance like that draws on the child's own formative powers and helps them flow again. Martina takes the brush, water and paint and has a go; and we see how happy she is by the expression on her face.

Space to come back to oneself

Children are often bombarded by too many powerful impressions. This can make them breathless, frantic, stressed and therefore hard to cope with

An expedition to a multiplex cinema is being planned for a nursery-age group in holiday childcare. 'It's just a film about fish, quite gentle,' says a member of staff. And yet these house-high pictures that rain down on you in quick succession are — in the true sense of the word — breathtaking.

Afterwards the children are over the top, and the walk back to the tube station is hard work. The exhausted carers exchange brief looks, and one has a sudden flash of inspiration: 'I noticed one fish in particular,' she says, 'and I'm going to paint it when we get back.'

'Do you mean the blue one with green stripes, and a kind of beard on its mouth?' asks one child. She makes a face that matches. 'I really liked that one. I'm going to paint it too.' The other children also calm down, and the painting session in the day-care centre brings them all back to themselves.

What is valuable about this, and can also apply to other circumstances? The carers opened a space which enabled the children to actively process and express the powerful impressions, and thus to come back to themselves. It's important that the adults involved did not just suggest something but also acted as examples.

9. Repose

A church concert. A father, mother and their four-year-old son are there. It's wonderful, surely, that the parents have taken their child with them to a special, peaceful place. But this boy has no idea about it being a place of quiet, because he behaves as though he's in the street. As if spring-loaded he rocks back and forth on the bench, stands up, runs about and makes a noise; and the father keeps talking at him. Finally he gives him his mobile phone to play with, then his wallet, which the child starts looking in. Small change clatters to the floor ...

Calm and quiet

What is lacking is repose: stopping for a moment, being calm, quiet and still. Children expect adults to help them to calm down — like these two children, who entered the church a little earlier.

At the entrance the father bends down to them and whispers something. The children look at him, look up at the beautiful high ceiling, look around them. Shining eyes, astonishment, whispers. No problem with quiet, for the father shows them how.

Quietening one's own voice is a little trick that experienced teachers use successfully. It can also help parents when we want to calm our children down.

Children want calm and quiet

A child to a nursery teacher who has just used her 'magic spell' to get the noise level down: 'Now it's nice again. When it's so loud we can't play properly.'

Similarly in a day-care centre: 'When can we eat lunch in your group again?' ask children from a different group. 'Why?' 'It's always so noisy in ours.'

And why is it so different? In that particular group, eating becomes an aesthetic experience too. Even if children only notice this subliminally, they behave more carefully if the dining table is arranged with more care. In this group the children help get the table ready each day: in the middle they put a small bowl with flowers they've picked themselves. And then there are rules: only one person can talk at a time.

And does this work? Well, of course sometimes children can't help interrupting, but each time they are told: 'Let him finish talking, then it will be your turn.' A nursery teacher reinforces this rule by placing her hand on that of the child who has interrupted. Being touched helps today's often restless children. It helps them feel perceived, addressed. The same thing is helpful at home too, if a child is restless at table. Give security by touching the child's arm: 'Stay sitting now.'

Touch calms

Touch is healing, calming and eases stress.

A mother reports, 'When my son used to come home from school he was always so wild. For the past couple of days I've been using this tip: when I greet him I stroke the nape of his neck a little, and somehow this does him good. This brief physical contact triggers something, like switching on a light.'

Tender skin contact is a form of active love which passes both physical and soul warmth to the other. This little boon also helps in the evening if it's proving hard to calm children down. When the child is in bed, try massaging his feet gently with a little lavender oil, first one foot, then the other. What's important here is your undivided attention: saying nothing for a couple of minutes, but just focusing on the child.

Movement

We often expect too much of children in asking them to be calm and quiet. For instance, we expect them to be quiet when we're talking to friends in a café. 'Be still now, or I'll put you in the high chair,' says a mother to a four-year-old who is just expressing his natural instinct to move.

It's also wholly inappropriate to ask children to be quiet and still if they are taken shopping for hours. Rebellion and restlessness is healthy in such circumstances, and ought to make us pause for thought: going shopping is stressful for children because it suppresses their natural joy in movement. Having to sit still for long periods — and in the midst of noise, adverts and a throng of people — is harmful for their life forces.

'Parking' them in front of the television is also disastrous. Artificial immobility not only hinders children's mental, emotional and physical development but also condemns them to 'inactivity stress.'

The fact is that children who haven't been able to rush around and let off steam during the day find it harder to fall asleep in the evening. We should reduce shopping trips with them to a minimum, and it's better to meet up with friends in a park where children can run about, climb, hop, balance and swing.

Where possible it's also good to take them out to the countryside (see also Chapter 10, p.113) and to protect them as much as possible from technical bombardment. Don't let them watch morning television, which nowadays makes teachers' work very difficult, since children are scarcely available for learning afterwards. Talk to each other instead of having the radio on at breakfast ...

Midday rest

If children come home in the middle of the day, they can have a rest after lunch. This is important for older children and essential for younger ones: they need this to recoup their energy. Quiet falls, no outer stimulus or artificial media: a little time out for everyone.

The child may not be able to sleep, nevertheless a quiet pause is important for coming back to oneself. You can make a rule that each person goes to his room for 'hush' time. Do something very quiet that no one else can hear: sleeping, resting, painting, looking at a picture book, reading — whatever ... The important thing is that each of us has a special time on our own to rest and recuperate.

'But I can't sleep!'

What can we do if a small child says, 'I can't sleep!'?

Give security — which we do by refraining from making the child our partner: no discussions, or any suggestion that a child should decide for himself. He can't yet (see Chapter 1, p.13). It's a good idea, instead, to take the child into his bedroom and have a little transition ritual.

'Now we're going to play the listening game,' says Dylan's mother to him.

'How do you play that?'

'We sit down very quietly. Hush. And now we listen out for everything that we can hear.'

Shutting our eyes makes it easier to hear things. Suddenly things are heard that would otherwise go unnoticed: the clock ticks, Dylan's tummy rumbles, the chair creaks, a bird twitters outside. Two minutes — and the child is calmer.

Then Dylan's mother says, 'Now I'm going to leave you to rest for half an hour.'

'How long is half an hour?'

Young children best understand this through images. You can agree a sign: 'Until the big hand has got to here.'

The rest should last at least half an hour, and if possible an hour.

Fairy tales

Every day we should make space for spending time with children with our full attention. This can include telling them fairy tales: an important island of calm can be provided by stories with an archetypal content such as those of Grimm.

In every family we need a fixed time at least once a week — we can even write it on our calendar — devoted to fairy tales. This is also a wonderful way in which fathers can get more involved.

Listening in peace

And how do we get children to really listen calmly and quietly? The path is via the ear: 'Now listen for a moment.' Play a note or two on a stringed instrument, a bell or a sounding bowl:[16] 'When you hear no sound again, then look at me, and that will be our sign that the story can begin.'

Islands of calm

The following is another helpful island of calm for a young child who is struggling to settle. I call it 'magic water.' Of course we get this ready together: sleeves are rolled up and a thick towel is placed on a firm stool. And now put a bowl on it, at least half full of hand-warm water. Place a cork or two in the water, a jam-jar lid, perhaps a small beaker. And now just let the child be ... Water has a magical effect, and brings children back to themselves in a trice. Of course it's important that you stay nearby and emanate calm too, for instance by reading peacefully. Now you'll be able to!

10. Religion

There is a new baby in a four-year-old's family. He asks to go and see her on his own for a moment. His mother says he may, but for safety's sake turns on the baby monitor. What she hears touches her deeply: 'Tell me about heaven,' says her son, 'you know I've been away from it so long, I can't really remember any more.'[17]

'Who made the world?'

Young children have a natural sense of connection with a world of spirit from which they come. Quite openly and innocently their questions urge us to 'reconnect' (one meaning of 'religion') with this reality.

'One day,' says the mother of a four-year-old, 'my little girl really brought me up short by asking where she was before she was born. Before I could reply she said, "In heaven. And while I was there I saw you all already."' Then she ran off as if this was the most natural thing in the world.'

Likewise five-year-old Gabriella asked, 'Who made God?' And after a moment she said, 'I know the answer: he was always there, because if someone had made him then he wouldn't be God.'

Magic moments

How many adults could easily answer such profound questions? Children give us these gifts if we stay open and attentive to them.

Just now, on a walk, Francesca asked out of the blue, 'Why am I a human being?' Then she stops to think: 'Yes, that's what you mean when you say "I" because that's always yourself. No one else can say it to you. Only I can say "I" to myself.'

Brief, magic moments give us a glimpse into the inner wealth of the child's world.

Children seek meaning, and unconsciously are passing through humanity's evolutionary stages.[18] That is why it's so important to pray with them. Saying an evening prayer to them in the cradle, and later saying one with them, is nourishment for the soul.

Children need this as much as their daily bread. 'I was lucky,' said the musician Albert C. Humphrey, 'my parents prayed.'[19]

Children feel deep satisfaction and security if they can sense that there is a higher reality they can turn to, and to which parents turn.

Being truthful

Children want to pray, but we can't meet this need with technical gadgets. If a teddy bear spools off a 'prayer' at the press of a button, or says that he will protect the child, this is a false message. Even if children don't show it, this will injure their feelings deeply. They have a fine sense for the fact that soul nourishment is something that only works between people. If a prayer is not something you can relate to, it's better to leave it altogether, for we must be honest with and in front of children. You could instead use a neutral, homely evening verse, such as this one:

> *Good mother night comes from the West*
> *Makes everything soft and dark:*
> *She seals each flower, and stills the lark*
> *And rocks the wild winds to rest —*
> *So now sleep gently too:*
> *Sleep deep, sweet dreams to you.*

What comes from the heart, reaches the heart. Children still have an intuitive sense of the power of a prayer or verse. If there's room for one in the morning, it can really make children shine with pleasure:

> *O sun, so golden in the sky*
> *Shine down upon me all the day*

> *Till everything I do and say*
> *Shines ever brighter back to you.*

After visiting another family, now that she's back at home and the family is about to start eating as usual, a four-year-old calls out, 'Pray first!' She took pleasure in the mood of the grace spoken in the other family.

Pausing for a moment before eating and sensing the family's togetherness in a shared moment of thanks can certainly create a healing space in busy family life.

Attentiveness and respect

Children like to see how a grown-up reacts when they do something.

On a school outing to the countryside, a child continually pulls the heads off flowers along the path. The teacher tells her to stop.

Another child asks, 'What's so bad about it?' The question shows that admonishments leave children inwardly untouched.

The teacher tries again, now with great presence of mind: she bends down to one of the torn-off flower heads and observes it carefully, admiring its colours and shape; she tells about the bees, bumble bees and butterflies that now won't be able to visit it. 'It makes me sad,' she says, 'if something beautiful like this is simply torn off and thrown away.'

'We can take them home with us and put them in water,' calls one of the children, who have all gathered round as though astounded at the seventh wonder of the world. One, then another and then many children bend down and gather up the fallen flowers.

Such an incident can show us what to do in other situations where a child injures something or someone. Respectful behaviour is only learned by example. As soon as we adults try to engage imaginatively with another person or creature in this way, the important sense that 'all life is sacred' awakens in children, as Albert Schweitzer so tellingly put it.

To teach children this is one of the most important tasks of education, for if we lose respect for living things we lose respect for ourselves as well.

Looking through God's window

In a big store, a mother says to her three-year-old, 'Go and play in the play corner if you like. I'm going to have a look around for a moment.'

She comes to fetch the child after two or three minutes, and then sees the giant screen which her child has been sitting in front of, spellbound. She takes her away, but at bedtime the child asks, 'Mum, how do you get pictures out of your head again?'

'Do you mean the pictures you saw today in the shop?' The child nods.

The mother thinks for a while and her gaze falls on a bunch of daisies that they picked on their last walk together. 'Now, I know something that always helps.' Expectant eyes gaze at her. 'The best thing is to look through God's window a little.' The next moment, these small, delicate flowers we usually don't give a second thought to, become a miracle: 'Look, no person on earth has ever made such a beautiful thing, and will never be able to.' Astonishment. 'The flowers look like tiny suns — yellow inside and with lots of rays all around.'

'The flowers are happy that we're looking at them, aren't they?'

'They certainly are. And now see if you can still see what they look like when you shut your eyes.' Lucy firmly shuts her eyes.

'Yes!' she says, beaming.

Children love to hear about goodness

'Dad, there are more good people than bad ones, aren't there?' asks a seven-year-old suddenly in a café.

Children want to hear about goodness: it is nourishing for them to hear about people who have ideals and who act on them. We can meet this need by telling them about modern heroes, of whom there are so many,[20] also close to hand. For instance, the neighbour's girl who, when she finished school, went abroad to help poor folk in a shanty town; or the friend who works as a nurse. It's great how children point us to what's important. Then, in a little article at the back of a newspaper, we might find reports of courageous contemporaries: wonderful food for conversation that broadens horizons and awakens courage and a positive mood.

Expanding horizons

Today, when external circumstances take up so much of our time, it's important to lead children consciously to what can give inner support. We can find this in nature, if we walk with children and discover wonderful things with them, and show our real astonishment and interest.

One unforgettable experience — though maybe only possible on holiday — is to go out with a child very early in the morning and wait for sunrise. Or go to the woods and place your ear against a tree trunk, and see what you can hear.

'No day passes without something special happening, that can give us joy ... we just have to open our eyes.'[21]

Art as umbilical cord

Art contains manifold possibilities. According to the famous conductor Nikolaus Harnoncourt, 'Art is not a nice extra — it is the umbilical cord which connects us to the divine, it guarantees our being human.' Small things can be important.

A young mother tells us, 'At home I've got a lovely art card of a painting by Raphael, called 'The Madonna and Child.' I put it up above the nappy-changing table so that I can look at it when I'm changing my baby's nappy. When I see the loving devotion in this picture, I feel myself affirmed as a mother, and it helps.'

There's a saying that goes, 'If you think of angels, their wings will spread.'

11. Regeneration

Once there was a king who ruled his land happily and wisely and looked after his people to the best of his ability. One evening, as he was playing dice, an important visitor was with him as a guest.

'Allow me to put a question to you,' said the visitor. 'You are so highly esteemed as a wise ruler, and now I see you are playing dice, just like the ordinary folk.'

'Well,' said the king, 'I'll tell you a secret. The human being is like a bow. To do good work you have to be strung and tense; but you will only achieve your goals if you let go occasionally.'

Looking after ourselves

This also applies to parents. Amidst all the duties, timetables and concerns for our children's welfare, we can forget about looking after ourselves. Yet it's true to say that what happens on the inside is reflected on the outside. If we are inwardly worn out and dissatisfied this will affect those around us and vice versa: the more composed the parents are, the happier their children will be.

Wish list

If we did have any free time, how would we use it? This is a key question. Ask yourself what you would most like to do regularly to recharge your batteries, then take ten minutes to write down as many ideas as possible: reading a good book, going to an art exhibition, singing in a choir, making music, painting, making pottery; getting more exercise, such as walking, jogging, or dancing; or drawing on inner sources of strength such as Goethe recommends, 'Read at least one good poem a day.'

Just by thinking of these possibilities, our good mood can return. We have taken the first step towards looking after ourselves.

The next thing to do, to realize one of these wishes, is to free ourselves from the belief that as parents we must continually orbit our child like a moon round a planet. Children don't respond with gratitude to continual micro-management — mollycoddling, entertaining, overseeing, monitoring and so on; instead they respond with unhealthy demands that just raise stress levels still further.

An important rule for daily life is: never do for children what they could do for themselves. Start this when they're infants, and then they will really enjoy imitating what parents can do.

A mother of two teenagers found this out too late: 'It was the biggest mistake of my life that I never got the children to help me when they were young. And now I go on and on at them. I have to ask a hundred times for every small thing.'

Delegate

If you have a partner, consider together when one of you could take over from the other. Many fathers withdraw in resignation because they find too often that 'I can't do anything right, so I might as well not bother.'

For us mothers, recharging ourselves is closely connected with the difficult matter of letting go and leaving our partners to do tasks such as making breakfast. Daily. Regularly. Entirely. And to do so without checking all the time if it's being done 'right.' The same applies at weekends. Take time off when, for instance, Dad takes the children out to buy food at the farmers' market, then cooks a meal with them, or takes them to the park. Note your free times in the calendar and stick to them. Use them for doing something for yourself from your wish list.

Time for your partner

If parents are asked, 'What are you doing to nurture yourselves?' or 'When did you last go out together on your own — to the cinema, a nice restaurant or a concert?' they often reply, 'If we go out we always take the children.' Ultimately this comes at too great a cost, for sooner or later it will damage your relationship. Both parents need proper, quality time together: just the two of them! Regularly. This includes going out somewhere at least every two weeks.

Daily care for yourself

Caring for ourselves helps us cope more calmly with daily life. Before the day begins try to have at least a few minutes regularly just for yourself, as a daily ritual: your own time for a prayer, meditation, or an observation exercise. If you do something like this regularly, it will make it more effective. One mother tells us, 'I draw strength from taking a few moments to focus on something beautiful — a flower, preferably a rose, or sometimes the leaf of a tree or a stone I picked up.' It is certainly true that resting our eyes on something gives us greater inner composure.

You can also look after yourself during the day. For instance you can sit down in your favourite place in the afternoon with a cup of tea and let your thoughts roam. Children learn from this example that they can sometimes just do things for themselves, on their own.

> 'This is my time now!'
> 'How long will it last?' asks Anna.
> 'Until I've drunk my tea.'
> 'When will you have drunk your tea?'
> 'When there's no more in the cup.'
> 'And then you'll come back?'
> 'Yes, then I'll come back.'

Unwinding in the evening

We need to unwind and prepare for a good night's sleep, which is the best way to regenerate. A nice little ritual for 'inviting' good sleep is a lavender footbath shortly before bed each evening: a large bowl with plenty of room for both feet, water at about 36°C (97°F), add a few drops of lavender essence (such as Weleda's

Lavender Bath Milk), place your feet in the bowl with a blanket or towel over your knees, and just enjoy it for ten minutes. Your breathing will calm and you will feel more relaxed. It's even more effective if you sit very still rather than reading the paper or turning on the radio. Diversions don't really renew us; we need to take our regeneration in hand intentionally. And it doesn't help if the atmosphere at home is stressful or strained.

Acting before tension gets too great

Sometimes we say something in a stressful situation which we regret afterwards. Later we feel guilty and promise ourselves not to say such things again. To ensure that, as far as possible, we don't do this, we can engage consciously in an activity that invokes one of the four elements: earth, water, air or light (fire). You may feel temperamentally more drawn to one or other of these.

> *Earth*: 'Earth' yourself by running up and down the stairs once. Or walk in the open air, swinging your arms well, for ten to twenty minutes. Movement rebalances the body and thus also our emotions.
> *Water*: Drink a whole glass of water in one go — this will give you a clear head again astonishingly quickly. The same is true if you roll up your sleeve and let cold water run over the pulse at your wrist.
> *Air*: Breathe deeply and slowly, as though against a small resistance — as if you were blowing up a balloon for instance — and count to four as you do so. Repeat this a few times. You will feel your tension fading.
> *Light*: Get out of the house and raise your face to the sky, absorbing and bathing in its light.

By looking after ourselves, we enhance our joy in life and sense of self. We are not so easily unsettled, we become more relaxed and those around us will suffer less from our moods. We develop greater equilibrium. It has hardly been put better or more succinctly than by Novalis: 'Balance can replace strength — and every person should be in balance, for that is the real nature of his freedom.'[22]

12. Reflection

One day, two parents turn to their rabbi for advice because of serious problems they are having in raising their child. They ask this wise man to suggest something they could do to help their son overcome his problems. The rabbi thinks for a moment and then looks at the parents in some surprise and says, 'It's not your child who needs to change, but you who must change first.'[23]

'Wait a moment; let me think'

Saskia's parents pass an ice-cream vendor. Saskia wants an ice cream — now, right away. Her father stops: 'One moment,' he says, 'I first have to think whether you can have one or not.' Saskia is immediately quiet, and remains so even when her father says, 'I don't want to buy you an ice cream at the moment because the weather's much too cold.' But why doesn't Saskia make a fuss at this point? Is she a particularly 'easy' or 'model' child? Definitely not. Yet her parents have simply decided to stop being controlled by their child's whims: 'We just couldn't do it any more.'

Taking a moment to stop and think frees us from fulfilling everything that children often demand so vehemently. She has to have these particular shoes, this T-shirt, these socks or this toy. Or she absolutely must have this particular friend to play straight after nursery or stay overnight with a friend. As parents we could list a long catalogue of such demands. So the next time one arrives, first breathe deeply and think, 'Do I actually want to do what my child is asking?' If not, it's better to say straight out, 'No, not now, because ...' without further discussion. There are so many more interesting things we can discuss with children than whether they can have something or not.

Do we talk to our children enough?

Children need people who like talking to them and do so with patience; lack of this contributes to the increasing number of 'late talkers' and speech development disorders. Let's just ask ourselves whether we really talk enough to our children, or whether we only spend about ten minutes a day talking to them, as is the common average. Clearly, this is too little. The capacity to speak can only develop if we talk to children a lot.

But parents often object: 'I've no idea what I'm meant to talk to my child about!'

Talk about everything that's happening at the moment. As Emmi Pikler has shown,[24] this can start with very young children and babies: as we look after them tell children what we're doing right now. Reflecting on a range of things with older children is something they love to do.

Reflecting with children

Children live in the midst of plenty today, and often don't know how ordinary, everyday things are connected with each other.

'What's that brown thing there?' asks a six-year-old who is watching her uncle digging in the garden.

The uncle says, 'Come with me.' In the kitchen he washes 'the brown thing' carefully, then takes a knife and cuts a finger-length piece and gives it to the girl. 'Now do you know?'

'Ah, chips!' she says. And for the first time she has learned what a potato is.

If we get children to help and join in from an early age (see Chapter 8, p.90) we prevent them growing up at one remove from reality. It is enriching and at the same time important to encourage a culture of questioning within the family, both stimulating and answering questions.

Encourage a culture of questioning

'In our family,' says a father, 'the most exciting conversations start at the breakfast table, especially at the weekend when we can take our time. We ask things such as: what, where, how? What's on the table in front of us and which country did it come from? The bananas? Where do they grow and how? The oranges? The sultanas in the muesli? How do they get to our country, and how do they reach the shop? What do they need to grow well and thrive? Where does the bread come from? What grains does it contain? How is it made? What is added to it, which spices or seasoning? Where do they come from? In our house the encyclopaedia is the most used book.'

Questions about things close at hand are interesting for us all. Reflecting on what is visibly before them gives pleasure to children. They form a connection to the world, and become more attentive and respectful. Their food even tastes better.

Acknowledgment

A mother tells us, 'My "Aha" experience came recently when my children — aged nine and eleven — were at home on their own in the afternoon one day. I had hardly got inside the door when I started in on them: "The shoes are in the middle of the corridor again. And the kitchen — what a mess: crumbs everywhere. And the dirty dishes still in the sink!"

'Suddenly my son stood there in front of me and said, "Relax! If you do, you might see that you're only focusing on what's wrong instead of saying what's OK for a change!" That made an impact on me and made me pause for thought.'

Let's think for a moment: isn't this true of us all too often? Imagine someone shows us the following sums:

$$12 + 3 = 15$$
$$18 + 13 = 31$$
$$9 + 14 = 25$$
$$18 + 46 = 64.$$

What is our response? We are likely to say that one of the answers is wrong, although we could equally well say that three are correct!

The same thing applies to raising children: we should immediately and tirelessly reflect back to children what is right, because how else can they learn? Children long to be seen; if they receive too little positive attention they will grow disruptive, which always gets attention. It's better to catch children when they're doing something right — every day — and praise them. They need that to thrive.

Acknowledgment is important. It strengthens from within and is therefore far better than any reward such as sweets. Children do something for us because they love us, in marked contrast to a promised reward that serves to 'repay' a child for her work or action.

Effort is what counts

Acknowledgment must be given the moment you notice something positive: 'Well done for buttering the bread yourself today.'

Specifically refer to what is giving you pleasure rather than just saying, 'Great!' For instance: 'I'm really pleased that you came home on time.' Or a pat on the back: 'It's great that you shared the chocolate you got from Uncle Roger with your sister.' Or, to start with, just mention tiny things that a child has managed, which used to be so difficult for her: 'You put your shoes in the right place today — well done!'

With every acknowledgment a child learns that she is on the right path; she grows a little more inwardly and is motivated to keep trying repeatedly until she succeeds.

At all events, effort is what counts! Effort leads to ability, as in learning to walk. Everyone has talent, but only effort makes something of it. A look of acknowledgment, a loving word and a smile encourage children to keep trying.

What did you enjoy today?

Seeing the good is a dynamic source of energy which we as parents and carers can draw on. A helpful way to nurture it is to look back on our day and try to identify three positive things that happened. It's easiest to do this shortly before going to sleep.

* What experience with my child gave me pleasure?
* What went well?
* What am I grateful for today?

Experience shows that everyone can find something that they enjoyed. Even parents who consider their child particularly 'difficult' start smiling after reflecting for a moment, as though the string of an instrument has been plucked: 'Yes, that went really well!' And that allows us to reconnect with that feeling of longing so much for our child, when she was newborn, in those first, magical moments. Love, warmth and tenderness flow again.

Don't put off being happy until tomorrow when quite simple, practical things can bring happiness back into our lives.

An Interview with Christiane Kutik

Doris Kleinau-Metzler: Frau Kutik, how did you become a parent advisor?

Christiane Kutik: I originally trained as an interior designer and very much enjoyed working in that field. And then, at the end of 1970, my two children were born — and everything changed. A familiar experience for all parents. Suddenly you think and see everything differently: which doctor shall I take my child to, what foods are healthy ...? I was also fascinated to see how children master skills by themselves: from first turning over onto their tummies through crawling to walking and speaking; and then their curiosity, their unbounded interest in the world around them. My children taught me to see the world anew: everything you pass becomes something special — the stone, snail shell or building site. The world is so exciting for young children, and it also became so for me when I took time and looked more closely. Yes, one needs time to develop a relationship with a child: attachment and empathy do not arise automatically at birth.

DKM: So how did you start coaching other parents? The term 'coaching' or 'consultancy' is one familiar in the world of business — managers getting professional support for instance. Why are parents today seeking support for daily life with their children?

CK: My experience from many conversations is that parents often don't know what a young child needs — for example, a clear sequence, a fixed structure to the day and certain rules and rituals. How should parents know this? They lack the experience passed on in extended families, and sometimes they are so bombarded by information from friends, self-help books and the internet that they can no longer see the most important thing: that parents are the key figures in their children's lives who must give them security — and free space. But it's also normal for things to get chaotic from time to time, though parents think things in their household are worse than in any other. Sometimes despairing parents call me because 'we never get through a morning without screams and anger, until we feel completely exhausted and we only just manage to get to the bus in time.' Some mothers only escape the stress of the morning once they arrive at work. But children also have an enormously tiring day in front of them — in a large group with many other children at nursery, kindergarten or school.

DKM: What practical help do you offer parents? Do you give tips about how to do things better?

CK: I don't make specific suggestions, as every measure has to suit the particular family. What's important is that parents are truthful and stand behind what they say. In discussions without the child present we work on a specific, acute problem. My first question to parents is always to ask them to describe something special that they experienced with their child today, something that really gave them pleasure for a moment. And they always find something! That forms the basis for the work, because often parents' pleasure in their child has dissipated in the daily chaos.

The second thing I ask parents is to describe a specific situation that causes them problems, such as what happens in the mornings.

I elaborate questions and guide parents to the path that is right for them. For instance, they start to see that 'it takes much too long in the mornings for the child between waking up and leaving the house.' Young children need a clear sequence where one thing follows another. We draw up a clear timetable for the mornings: when a child is woken, goes to the bathroom, and a consistent place and time for a child to get dressed. It is not enough to tell young children 'Get dressed now!' To begin with they still need help and supervision. This also means that I as adult am really present. This doesn't work if I call out an instruction to a child and at the same time quickly fill the washing machine or have a phone conversation.

DKM: Children often get used to dawdling and drifting, and parents find it difficult to become suddenly strict. How, in your experience, can a timetable or plan help change this?

CK: One can establish new habits. Tangible change is always possible if one really tackles a problem. Often parents are on edge because it takes three quarters of an hour for a child to get dressed. One can decide on a helpful sequence and also precise times. It takes a while for good habits to become established. A key point that parents need to know in order not to give up after three days is that it will initially take four weeks to get new habits established; and then, preferably, a further four weeks to consolidate them. Of course it's important to be really clear. Clarity is the backbone of raising children. This has nothing to do with rigid strictness, but with giving a child security and stability.

DKM: The image of the 'backbone' for the necessary consistency seems very fitting to me, for a spine is not rigid either, but flexible — yet retains its form.

CK: Yes, this is the key approach. This means firstly taking on our role as parents in a quite clear and definite way. We parents are not the child's partner or friend. If I act as a friend: 'Would you like to eat this or that? Do you want to go out to play?' and so on, the child has no stability and no clear sense of what is good and right. We overtax children if we continually ask them to make decisions they are not yet mature enough to make, and which therefore cause them stress. Clarity of roles also means that I am clear what values are important in my family, because children need values. They don't have these as a given.

DKM: What do you mean by values? Parents often only gradually find their direction.

CK: I see values as something very practical, for example, that we eat with a knife and fork, start a meal together, don't crumble our food up into little pieces or bite into one biscuit and then another without finishing the first. However, this also involves not allowing ourselves to be insulted, or have our feelings injured — not even by our young children. Behaviour that still seems funny in a two-year-old becomes a problem in a six-year-old. Clarity of roles and respect are closely linked. Respect is not innate: this is something they learn through guidance and instruction. If an infant knocks his father's glasses off his nose, this isn't necessarily 'cute.' One can hold his hand back gently, and simply say, 'The glasses belong on Dad's nose.' A no must be a genuine no. The precondition for respectful interaction is that we parents first of all have self-respect, instead of going to enormous lengths to 'please the child.' Giving children guidelines also means valuing ourselves as parents and taking time and space for ourselves.

DKM: But parents also have a great deal of understanding for their children's behaviour: the child might be teething, or in a rebellious phase, or maybe has had problems with the child next door and so on ...

CK: Parents today tend to talk and interpret a lot. Do I really know exactly what's going on in a child? For instance, during the 'terrible twos' it's especially important to maintain a clear stance so that the child sees he can rely on his parents. Children need a safe harbour.

DKM: Yet there are repeatedly situations in which daily life is stressful and demanding for parents.

CK: Our way of life often makes children restless. Young children don't have to be carted around everywhere: they still need a lot of sleep, and they need space to explore, experiment, move around in the open air and play. Few but good quality toys stimulate play better than a whole pile of things that the child has to make continual choices about. And every mother and father — whether working or not — needs a clear structure to their day so that children know what's happening and can rely on it as the basis for their own lives. By nature children live in the moment, and if something occurs to them they want to do it here and now. Children can teach us about living in the present: for example, in a stressful situation we can get them to leap into a different 'now' if we offer them something tangible. We might take a few steps to the window and say, 'Oh, look at that tiny dog going by ...' or 'Wait a moment, I must just turn the kettle off.' Such tiny things are surprisingly helpful for alleviating stressful situations. The decisive thing is to manage the demands on us with composure.

DKM: In other words, instead of arguing with a grumpy child, we can offer him a different situation. But the composure you're talking about is particularly difficult during stressful moments.

CK: Naturally, maintaining equanimity and composure can be problematic for all of us. It's a path you decide to pursue. In a stressful situation it's always helpful to stop for a moment, breathe deeply and ask, 'Do I actually want to do what the child is demanding so insistently?' By doing this we perceive ourselves and observe how we react in critical situations. Of course, parents wish to do everything right, but it's normal to make mistakes and no one should feel guilty if they do. We can reflect on the situations that are difficult for us — and then take the next step, and the next. It's an exciting journey, and rewarding because it will gradually make daily life less stressful, and allow joy and pleasure to return.

This interview first appeared in *a tempo*, the lifestyle magazine produced by the the two publishing houses Verlag Freies Geistesleben and Urachhaus.

References and Notes

1 Anne Jean Ayres
2 Jacques Lusseyran
3 Bernhard of Clairvaux
4 Janusz Korczak
5 Martin Large
6 Anne Jean Ayres
7 *Der Stern*, no. 22, May 21, 2008
8 Horst Eberhard
9 Hilde Domin, 'Es gibt dich' from *Gesammelte Gedichte*
10 Eckhard Schiffer
11 See, for example, www.wellsphere.com/parenting-article/
    tv-viewing-causes-lag-in-infant-language-development/699102?que
    ry=Delayed+Language+Development
12 Alice Miller
13 Joachim Bauer
14 Alexander Mitscherlich
15 Anna Jean Ayres
16 See: www.soundingbowls.com
17 Bear Heart
18 Translator's note: this idea is based on the 'maturationist'
    theory of G. Stanley Hall, which posits that growing children
    recapitulate evolutionary stages of development as they grow up
    and that there is a correspondence between childhood stages
    and evolutionary history.
19 Spoken by the singer Albert C. Humphrey during an event in
    Munich in 2006.
20 William J. Bennett
21 Pablo Casals
22 Novalis
23 Armin Krenz (Ed.) *Handbuch für Erzieherinnen* (loose-leaf
    periodical) 06/2005 issue
24 Emmi Pikler, Anna Tardos

Bibliography

Ayres, Anne Jean (2005) *Sensory Integration and the Child*, Western Psychological Services, US.

Barz , Brigitte (1987) *Festivals with Children*, Floris Books, UK.

Bauer, Joachim (2006) *Warum ich fühle was du fühlst: Intuitiv Kommunikation und das Geheimnis der Spiegelneurone*, Heyne Verlag, Germany.

Bennett, William J. (1997) *The Children's Book of Heroes*, Simon & Schuster, US.

Bom, Paulien & Huber, Machteld (2009) *The Toddler Years: Growth and Development from 1 to 4 Years*, Floris Books, UK.

Casals, Pablo (1981) *Joy and Sorrows*, Eel Pie Publishing, UK.

Clairvaux, Bernhard of; Dollen, Charles (Ed.) (1996) *On the Love of God and Other Selected Writings*, Alba House,US.

Domin, Hilde (1999) *Gesammelte Gedichte (7th edition)* S. Fischer, Germany.

Eberhard, Horst (1975) *Friedrich der Staufer*, Claassen Verlag, Germany.

Goebel, Wolfgang; Glöckler, Michaela (2007) *A Guide to Child Health*, Floris Books, UK.

Grimm; illustrated by Anastasiya Archipova (2000) *Favourite Grimm's Tales*, Floris Books, UK.

Heart, Bear (1998) *The Wind Is My Mother: The Life and Teachings of an American Shaman*, Berkley Books, US.

Jones, Michael (Ed.) (1996) *Prayers and Graces*, Floris Books, UK.

Kiel-Hinrichsen, Monika (2006) *Why Children Don't Listen: A Guide for Parents and Teachers*, Floris Books, UK.

Korczak, Janusz (2007) *Loving Every Child: Wisdom for Parents*, Algonquin Books, US

Kornberger, Horst (2008) *The Power of Stories: Nurturing Children's Imagination and Consciousness*, Floris Books, UK.

Large, J.; Carey, D. (1998) *Festivals, Family and Food,* Hawthorn Press, UK.

Large, Martin (2003) *Set Free Childhood: Parents' Survival Guide for Coping with Computers and TV,* Hawthorn Press, UK.

Lockie, Beatrys (2010) *Bedtime Storytelling: A Collection for Parents,* Floris Books, UK.

Lusseyran, Jacques (1985) *And There Was Light,* Floris Books, UK.

Miller, Alice (1990) *For Your Own Good: Hidden Cruelty in Child-rearing and the Roots of Violence,* Farrar Straus Giroux.

Mitscherlich, Alexander (2008) *Die Unwirtlichkeit unserer Städte,* Suhrkamp Verlag Kg, Germany.

Novalis; Margaret Mahony Stoljar (Ed.) (1997) *Philosophical Writings (Fragments)* State University of New York Press, US.

Oliver, Jamie (2001) *Happy Days with the Naked Chef,* Michael Joseph, UK (contains a very informative chapter with ideas for cooking with children).

Pikler, Emmi; Tardos, Anna (2005) *Miteinander vertraut warden. Erfahrungen und Gedanken zur Pflege von Säuglingen und Kleinkindern,* Arbor Verlag, Germany.

Schiffer, Eckhard (1999) *Warum Huckleberry Finn nicht süchtig wurde. Anstiftung gegen Sucht und Selbstzerstörung bei Kindern und Jugendlichen,* Beltz, Julius, Germany.